SPIKE UP!

BECOMING AN ATHLETE AT 60

Jeanne Roy

Spike Up!

Copyright © 2023 by Jeanne Roy.

All rights reserved. No part of this publication may be reproduced, distributed, or transmitted in any form or by any means, including photocopying, recording, or other electronic or mechanical methods, without the prior written permission of the publisher, except in the case of brief quotations embodied in critical reviews and certain other noncommercial uses permitted by copyright law.

The contents of this book include stories, situations, conversations, and information relying on the memory of the author alone. Any mistakes or misquoting are that of the author alone.

For permission requests, write to Jeanne Roy at bodyindependent@gmail.com

Spike Up! / Jeanne Roy —1st ed.
ISBN 979-8-218-20159-3

Cover photo by Danny Harris

CONTENTS

Spike Up!

For Dean, my cutman for life. Wut?

Spike Up!

This book is for everyone who has wanted to do something but was afraid. Afraid it would hurt physically, afraid it would hurt emotionally, afraid that people wouldn't understand or, worse, wouldn't care. Afraid that after putting your heart, mind, body, and soul into something, you, by your own definition, would fail; not only in your eyes, but in the eyes of others as well.

No matter what the motivational posters say, it's scary to put yourself out there, to open yourself to criticism, even ridicule. It's much easier to do nothing and therefore, risk nothing. But you know what? Some people are going to like and support what you do and some won't. Do you like, understand, or even care, about what every person on this earth is doing? Of course not. We're all different. Just keep in mind that the only people who are going to want to hurt you are those who don't have the guts to do what you are doing.

Spike Up!

In today's world, we're bombarded with stories about ageism, sexism, ism, ism. We're told, if you're a woman, a man, however you identify, over 50, 60, 70, you're repressed, depressed, ignored, and disregarded. Don't listen to them. I didn't. Instead, I stepped into a gym, onto a track, and onto an obstacle course. Sometimes scared, sometimes confident, sometimes feeling like an idiot, sometimes all three and then some. You want to know what happened? <u>Every single time</u>, I encountered kindness and support. To this day, the focus isn't on how strong or how fast I am. What really matters is that I show up, do the work, give my best. If I do that, the results will speak for themselves.

Are you ready to show up, do the work, give your best? This is not a "how to" book; I can't teach you how to make that decision, but if you need a little encouragement or some inspiration, read on, and by the time you are finished, you'll be ready to "Spike Up!" and make it happen.

I am an Athlete

Walking out onto the track, I stand behind the blocks, and wait for the Starter to give the commands.

"On your marks"

I step up and press my feet into the blocks, fingers at the line shoulder width apart. My body is ready. My mind is ready. I know what I need to do.

"Set"

My mind empties, I lean forward and raise up. There is nothing but me and the track.

"Bang!" The gun fires.

I explode out of the blocks, arms swinging loose and strong, spikes pounding into the track. Practice becomes performance. Approaching the finish line, the only thing I hear is Coach yelling at the top of his lungs "Finish it counselor! Finish it!"

I do. I finish it. I am 61 years old.

I am an athlete.

Spike Up!

CHAPTER ONE

Setting the Course

Although born in Southgate, California, my memories begin in the house in Garden Grove where we moved when I was around 3 years old. I didn't know it then, but my upbringing was unusual in that my father, due to a heart condition, stayed home while my mom went to work. As a "stay-at-home dad" working without a template, he focused on what he thought were important skills. These included riding a tricycle and bicycle, as well as more creative skills such as blowing bubbles with bubble gum, and using said bubble gum on the end of a broomstick to get things that fell through the floor heater. Lest my intellect go unchallenged, he taught me how to identify the states by their shape and baseball teams by their cap. Even at a very young age, it was clear the direction I was headed.

Spike Up!

My mother tried to change that direction and
repress the tomboy in me by enrolling me in tap
and ballet classes. Unfortunately, for my mom
anyway, I wasn't interested in the ballet part.
Who wants to tip toe in slippers when you can
clack, clack, clack in tap shoes? Maybe this was
my mother's underhanded way of developing
my (stereotypical female) love of shoes, in
which case, she succeeded. The dance class
thing lasted until I was about 8. I don't recall
why it ended, so it obviously wasn't a traumatic
event.

Shortly thereafter, we moved to Anaheim where
I could indulge in running, jumping, and
hanging upside down from whatever was
available, trees, monkey bars, the side of the
bed. Continuing my "education," my dad taught
me the basics of bat, ball, and glove, installed a
tether ball court in the driveway, and, deciding
that a bicycle wasn't good enough for "his little
girl," bought me a unicycle. I learned to ride the
darn thing and still have the scars to prove it.

It might have been the unicycle that prompted mom to try again, this time with baton twirling. How she came up with that idea, I will never know. In any event, off I went to become part of the Anaheim Warriors baton twirling team. The connection between twirling a baton and being a warrior was a bit tenuous, the uniforms even more so, but what the heck, it was the 70s. And what says 70s better than a gold top and shorts, leopard gauntlets and black cowboy hat, or a red sequined leotard with a Russian-style feather hat? Boots! Black knee-high boots!

Baton twirling was more my style. Throwing the baton high enough to be able to spin three times and catch it before it hit the ground was exhilarating, as was twirling a fire baton (and no, it doesn't burn if it hits you). The fire baton was for the Fireman's Parade where I was able to have my regular baton autographed by Grand Marshalls Kevin Tighe and Randolph Mantooth, stars in the television show *Emergency!* I really should have kept that baton. There also was the whistle. Somehow, I became a squad leader and squad leaders were given whistles so they could issue commands to the twirlers. In my first competition as a squad leader, we won the Sweepstakes trophy. What stands out in my mind, however, is marching up to the presenter to the song Hey Big Spender, which I now realize was totally inappropriate for an 11-year-old, and the zipper on the back of my uniform coming apart. Being a future Miss Poise, I kept on smiling and collected the trophy. Somewhere out there is a whistle with my name on it. I should have kept that too. Baton twirling also gave me my first sports related injury. A fellow twirler was swinging her baton by the tip (not a good idea) and lost control. Unfortunately, my face was in the path. Dad came to the rescue with a bag of frozen peas.

Entering Trident Junior High in 1972 freed me from my mother's efforts in "redirection," but looking back, I must have understood that being a tomboy at home was one thing, but how I behaved at school was another. There were girls' sports at my school, but no one encouraged me in that direction. It probably didn't help that I was younger and smaller than all my classmates, as well as shy and introverted. Even though we engaged in sports in Physical Education class, I didn't see organized sports as something that involved me. (Title IX, which prohibits sex-based discrimination in any school or any other education program that receives federal funding had just been passed, but it would be 10 years or more before it would have any real effect.) My dad watched sports on TV and we watched the Olympics, but no one in my world was an athlete. My crowning achievements were being named Miss Poise by the faculty and being selected to join Block T, the pep squad. At least I was starting to break out of my shyness shell and I did get to wear 1970's style saddle shoes with my blue and white dress. In retrospect, it probably was the shoes that convinced me to try out in the first place. It certainly wasn't the dress

1975 brought me to Loara High School which brought me closer to being an athlete. At Loara, (home of the Saxon Marching Band and Valkyrie Drill Team) the drill team was a big deal. In case you were wondering, one of the myths surrounding the Valkyrie is as "chooser of the slain" she would guide souls of the dead into Valhalla. Wish I'd have known that then!

Tryouts involved learning a dance routine, learning to march, and learning to perform in front of judges. I would never have tried out on

Spike Up!

my own, but my friends were trying out, so I went along. I was the only one selected. Go figure. (My friends would join me the following year)

As a member of the Drill Team, I marched in parades carrying a sword and shield, and performed during half-time at football games wearing a sequined top hat and tails. With both uniforms, I wore silver marching boots with red tassels – very stylish, but extremely uncomfortable (high heels anyone?) and bearing no resemblance, I'm sure, to anything the Valkyrie would have worn.

In addition to wearing stylish outfits, Drill Team introduced me to the concept of training. We learned dance routines during the summer, and the week before school started meant being on the field from 8 to noon, Monday through Friday. Once school started, we were on the field before school and through first period which was Physical Education AKA Drill Team. We hit the field after school and finished when it started to get dark.

Our coach, Mrs. A. was a taskmaster who brooked no nonsense. As far as she was concerned, we were there to be champions. Period. Not 3rd, 2nd, or 1st. It was Sweepstakes or nothing, and if you weren't willing to do the work, "don't let the door hit you on the way out." When I tell people about my experiences with Drill Team, most respond with "Oh my gosh!" or "That's horrible!" Mrs. A. was never cruel or mean. She set the bar high and gave us the chance to learn the skills necessary to get over it. She demanded excellence in training and in performance. She told us "You should never lose points at inspection," meaning that if something was within our control, we were responsible for the outcome. Mrs. A. taught us how to be champions.

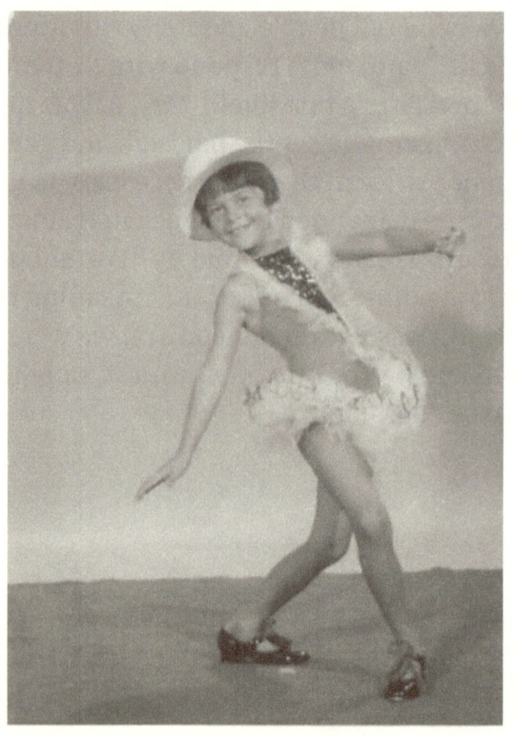

A dancer's pose

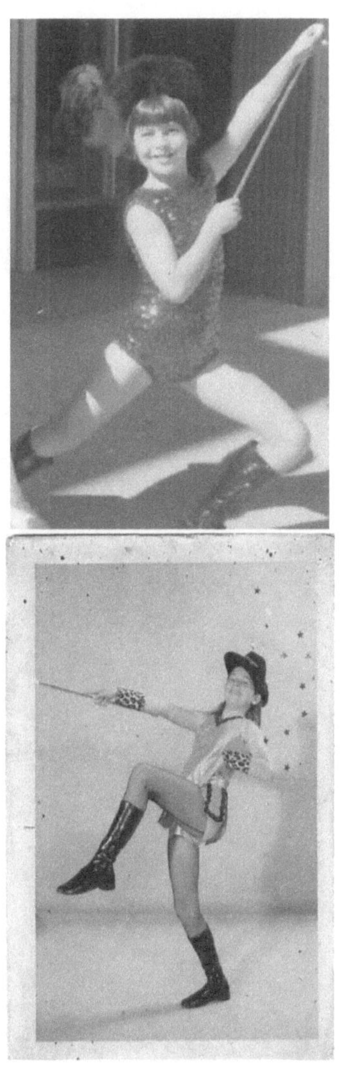

The boots make the outfits

Spike Up!

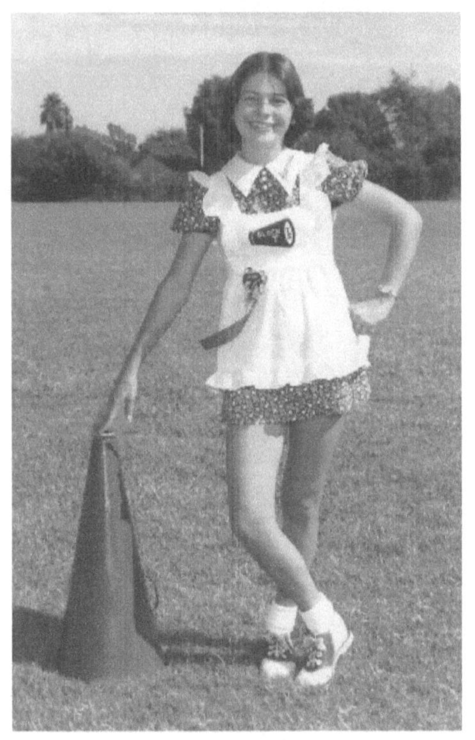

Go Dolphins!

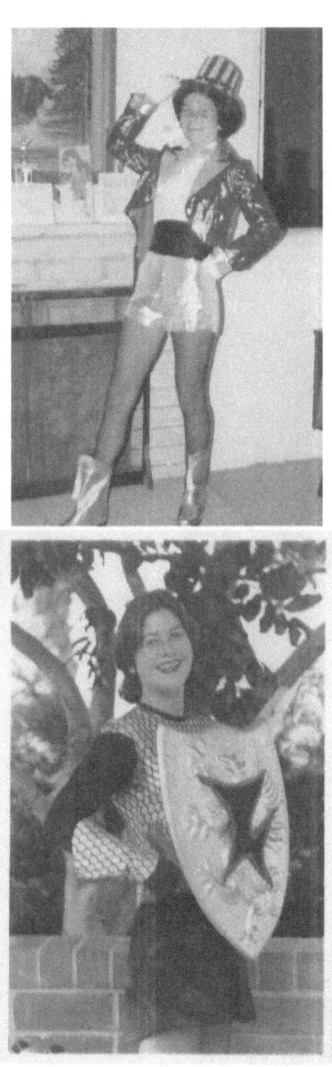

Ride of the Valkyries

Spike Up!

CHAPTER TWO

Muscling Up

The fitness revolution was just beginning when Holiday Health Spa (which would become Bally Total Fitness and then LA Fitness) opened near my house. A friend suggested we check it out. In minutes I was hooked; not by the classes, not by the machines, not by the track, not by the pool, but by the weights. Dumbbells, barbells, all shiny and organized on their racks calling "lift me, lift me." I didn't know a thing about lifting weights, I just knew that it was something I wanted to do. Fortunately, there were separate weight rooms for men and women with the women's space a wasteland just waiting to be industrialized by the few of us looking to build. But how? And what to wear?

Spike Up!

This was long before the internet, so there were no YouTube videos to show you how to do a biceps curl, deadlift, or squat; there were no personal trainers. There was no Lululemon or Gymshark. What existed were a few books, all written by and for men, and Jane Fonda "Feel the Burn" workout video tapes. I found a book with simple instructions and clear pictures for the "how" and high-top Reeboks, footless white tights, white T shirt, covered with a baby-blue tank-style, thong leotard for the "wear." Alas, neither the book nor the pictures survive.

As these were the college years, time was my friend. With book in hand, and Reeboks on my feet, the weight room was mine. I would look at the pictures and try to mimic the movements. I didn't understand much about sets and reps so I just did some of everything. I loved everything about it. The feel of the weights in my hands, the way my muscles moved; when I lifted the weights, I felt powerful. Every now and again, someone would say something like "nice form" or "good job." Even though they probably didn't know any more than I did, you would think I had died and gone to heaven. Someone thought I was doing something right.

Things became more challenging when, in 1983, I moved to San Diego to attend law school. Time was no longer my friend. I had some weights, the kind with rubber plates that you could take on and off, but they were cumbersome to carry around as well as to use. My gym membership transferred, but it wasn't convenient, so I rarely went. My muscle tone faded and as I approached the end of my third year, between work and school, eating became an afterthought causing me to drop to an unhealthy weight. It was only after my friends staged an intervention that I even noticed how gaunt I had become. This lesson in paying attention to my body would become more important as the years passed.

After law school, I embarked upon what would be a 30+ year career with the Riverside County District Attorney's Office. How much time I spent in the gym was in direct correlation to my assignment at the time. Some assignments left little free time, others more so. Even though I still loved lifting weights (I even bought a weight belt, which I still have and still wear), it wasn't a priority. I tried getting up early and working out at home, going to the gym at lunch, or going to the gym after work. I was either too

Spike Up!

tired, the gym was too crowded, or I was too busy. I didn't have a weight problem and was able to do whatever I wanted to do, so going to the gym became something I still did, but not with any regularity, until I hit 48.

I was standing in a store check-out line behind two women who were discussing what they had done for their 50th birthdays. Both were extremely overweight and what they considered a great birthday was my idea of hell. I went home and told my husband we were joining the local gym. (Shout-out to Foothill, now Ultraflex, gym in Monrovia, CA) That was my first turning point; the second would come 10 years later.

Even though I was still working and with an hour-long commute each way, the gym was now a priority. My routine became established. I came home, let the dogs out, changed my clothes, fed the dogs, and went to the gym. Any disruption in my routine risked failure, so with rare exception, I didn't deviate.

Being an introvert by nature, saying "hi" to people at the gym was as close as I came to making friends. My husband, on the other hand, got to know the owner, the staff, the trainers, and many of the members. With my husband as the lead, I could slip in the back door and become friends by association. It served me well as I then developed my own relationships, especially with Carlos, who would become my personal trainer after my second turning point arrived at the end of 2018, almost with a bang.

There are two pillars in front of our garage, and what better to have on a pillar than a planter? A heavy, ceramic, funnel-shaped planter, with colorful trailing flowers. My husband had put the planters up but they needed to be replanted. I wanted to take them down and clean them out before replanting. Taking them down wasn't much of a problem, putting them back up was another story. Standing on the ladder, I went to put the planter back up on the pillar and with about 2 inches to go, realized I was in trouble and that this was going to end one of three ways. I was going to drop the planter, the planter and I were both going to hit the ground, or I was going to get the planter up on the pillar. With options one and two being unacceptable, I used every ounce of strength I had to lift the planter and get it those last 2 inches up onto the pillar. Arms and legs shaking, I climbed down the ladder and said to myself "never again." Not "never again" to lifting a planter but "never again" to not being able to. I met with Carlos that week and have never looked back, not even when the world changed in 2020.

When the government shut down the gym, we took our gym to the park where we would stay for the next 18 months. Between Carlos and his clients, we put together enough equipment to do what we needed to do. We had weights, bands, steps, a portable bike and a stair stepper. Some of us (including Karen, who I will blame for many of my ills) became part of the "Quaranteam" and did the Friday Fitness Course which involved sled pulling, running, jumping and other exercises, all against the clock. It was great. We weren't the only people out there and Carlos made friends with all of them and, by association, so did the rest of us. The guys who worked at the park kept us up with the local gossip; we knew the walkers, the runners and the bocce ball players. We knew the yoga ladies and the people who set up their orchestra in the afternoon. We made friends

with all the dogs, usually knowing their names
before those of their owners. We were a kind of
family. We trained in the heat and the cold, the
wind and rain. I got into the best shape of my
life with a great tan as a bonus. I also learned to
run.

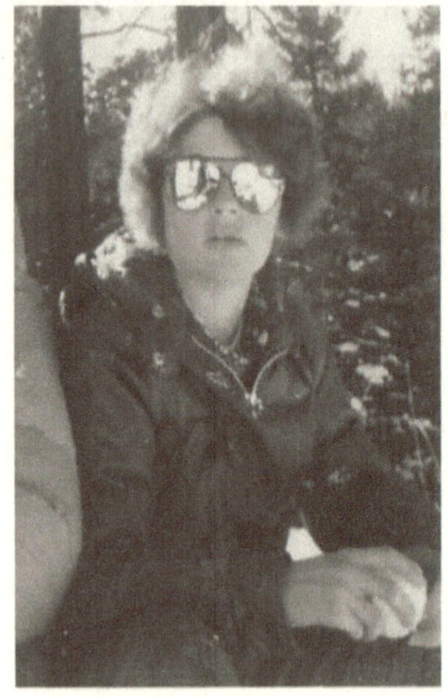

College cool

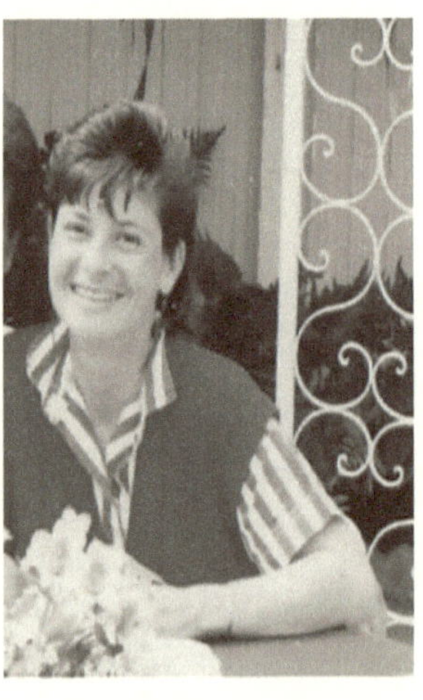

A little too thin

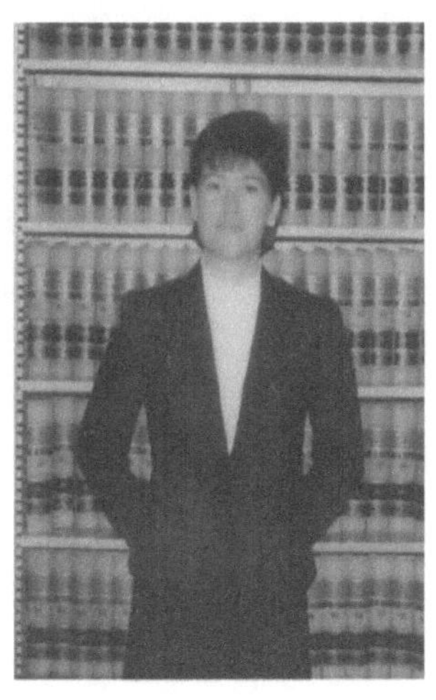

Law Clerk 1988

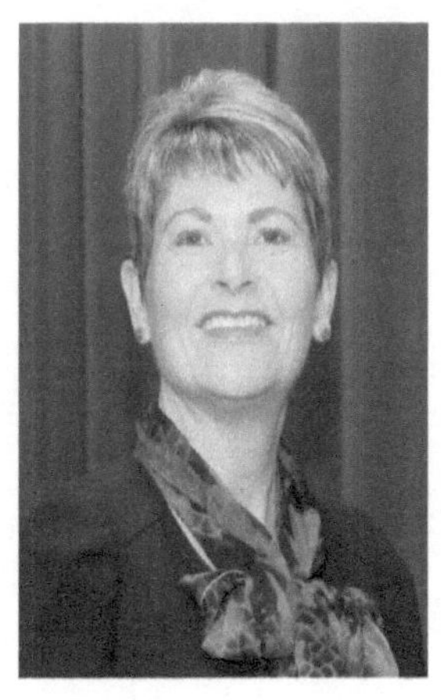

Assistant District Attorney 2018

Spike Up!

CHAPTER THREE

Just One Lap

I hate running. I hate everything about it. I hate the slap of my feet on the pavement. I hate squinting into the sun with sweat dripping down my back. I hate the cold on my face and in my hands.   What I do love is being able to run, how good I feel when it's over and wearing really cool shoes.

It started with just one lap at the park, about a third of a mile. Carlos decided that part of our new training regimen would include running. You have got to be kidding me? You want me to do what? Ok, fine, I'll do one lap. How hard can it be? I thought I was going to die right there on the pavement in the middle of the park. Maybe they would erect a monument "She died trying." At least it would have been over. An hour of

Spike Up!

whining later, I did one more lap. And so it went, more whining, more laps. It seemed my body was going to become that of a runner, whether I liked it or not.

As with most things, I figured if I was going to run, I might as well learn something about it. This time, I had the internet at my disposal and read article after article. I ordered books on running anatomy, science, technique, injury prevention. I read books about runners, marathoners, ultra-runners, all of which confirmed my belief, one which I still hold, that those people are insane.

The more I ran, the more I hurt. From below the knees down, I was a wreck. I became convinced it was my shoes and embarked upon a quest to find the perfect running shoe. Foot shape, arch position, pronate, supinate, heel strike, cushioned, flat, road, trail, the options were endless. After I tried every one of them with no success, my husband, who watched all this with some amusement, said "Your foot strike is off." What? Seriously? My foot strike? You mean the answer isn't another pair of running shoes?

(Darn) Why didn't you say something? "Would you have listened?" Uh, well. As always, he was correct about both the foot strike and me (not) listening. Enter the second coolest thing about running, K-tape. KT TAPE, kinesiology therapeutic tape, is that stuff you see on all sorts of athletes. They tape their shoulders, arms, legs, you name it. It creates stability which can decrease pain. I bought some in hot pink because, well, it was hot pink, and because the part of wearing K-tape that no one mentions, is that you want other people to see how cool you are "working through the pain." Except that once my husband taped me up, there was no pain! I almost cried; not because there was no pain, but because now I could buy shoes just for the cool factor. Running was not going to be a waste after all. Wearing the tape trained me (and my feet) how to run properly. Eventually, the tape came off and I could, and still can, run without pain. People look at me and assume I'm a runner. I still don't like running but I love being able to run. I also have a collection of very cool running shoes.

Spike Up!

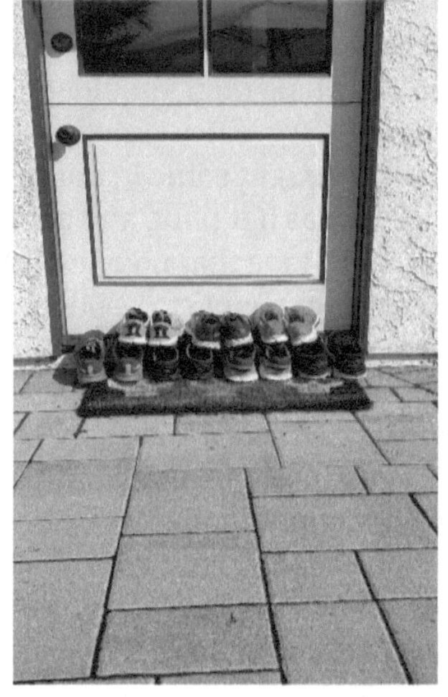

What remains from the grand experiment

CHAPTER FOUR

Only 50 Meters

For this part to make sense, we have to back up to when I started training with Carlos. When I was thinking of working with a personal trainer, I looked around the gym to see with whom I might be a good fit. I wanted someone who would make me work. I knew Carlos and knew he really trained his people. I told him about the planter incident and what I was hoping to achieve. We set up a schedule and got started. Nothing I had done before prepared me for this. I knew I was on the right track when my husband told me that one of the other trainers had pulled him aside and said "He's training her like she's 22!" My husband, being who he is, responded "Well, she's getting home ok. Maybe I should slip him an extra twenty." Carlos and I thought that was hilarious; I'm pretty sure the price went up.

The early days were rough. The first time I did wall squats, I almost passed out. Who knew your blood could pool in your feet so quickly? Carlos had me sit down and drink about an ounce of some concoction that tasted like what I imagine cough syrup would taste like if you mixed it with motor oil. It did the trick. Not only did it get me back on my feet, but motivated me to keep working because I was never going to drink that sludge again. I trained twice a week with one day for upper body and the other for lower. Our focus was on strength, so I did a lot of heavy lifting but never more than I could handle. Even though I loved training, I would occasionally resort to whining. One day when I was whining that I was tired, Carlos simply looked at me and said "You know, you wouldn't be so tired if you stopped rolling your eyes." I laughed so hard I almost cried. It must have taken me 10 minutes to recover. And on it went.

Spending serious time in the gym allowed me to think about the gym more seriously. I started looking around and noticed that, at least when I was there, I didn't see many older people lifting. Maybe a couple of men, but no women that were doing what I was doing. Occasionally, an older woman would say something like "You're amazing" or "I could never do that" which I thought was odd, as I was no one special. I just showed up and did the work.

It will come as no surprise that I started researching older adults and physical fitness. Most of it reinforced the notion that you get old, "fall, break a hip, end up in a home and then you die." It's always all four. There was no scenario where, because you were strong, you didn't fall. You never fall and bruise your elbow. You never fall, break a hip and recover. You only "fall, break a hip, end up in a home and then you die." As far as I could tell, that threat was used to sell products and give people excuses to not do anything they didn't want to do. The "Senior Fitness" classes I saw seemed to be of the same mindset, preaching "Just do what you can," "Don't push yourself," "Take it easy." I wondered how, over the years, we went from "Go for it" "You can do it" "Keep going" to

Spike Up!

essentially being one with the couch. I didn't like what I saw. I kept digging.

As with most things, once you know what you are looking for it becomes easier to find. I started seeing articles about women and men in their 80s, 90s, 100s who were active and engaged. For obvious reasons, the women stood out. There were women in their 90s swimming, doing yoga, and gymnastics. There were women in their 70s, 80s, and 90s running 5ks, marathons, and triathlons. And then there was Julia "Hurricane" Hawkins who, in November of 2021, at 105, would run the 100-meter dash at the Louisiana Senior Games.

I discovered Ms. Hawkins in 2020 and as a result, the Senior Games. State Senior Games are open to anyone 50 or older and have numerous sports in which athletes can compete. To participate in the National Senior Games, you must qualify in your sport at a qualifying Senior Games. My thought process went something like this, "If a 105-year-old can do it, I can do it." and "No matter how bad it is, it will only last a few seconds." Not exactly a champion's mindset but it got me to say the words out loud, "I'm going to be a sprinter."

One problem was I didn't know anything about sprinting. I thought it was just running fast. Little did I know that running fast is the result of intense technical training. Another problem was I didn't have access to a track. What I did have was Carlos (who had a track and field background), starting blocks, and YouTube. My plan was to spend 2021 training with the goal of qualifying in 2022 and, hopefully, competing at Nationals in 2023. The best laid plans and all that.

We went back to the gym in the summer of 2021. Because we had spent the last 18 months at the park, I wasn't faced with losing weight or getting back into shape. I was in the best shape of my life. We had been doing "off and on" sprint training at the park and I was able to work some on starts on the turf area of the gym. We were able to get access to a track, but our schedules were such that regular practice wasn't possible. This wasn't a problem as qualifying games in California weren't until September

Spike Up!

2022, so we had plenty of time, until Carlos decided otherwise. San Diego had their yearly games in September of 2021. I made the mistake of mentioning it to Carlos who asked if I had registered. When I said there was no way I could be ready, he simply gave me his look and said "If you wait until you are ready, you'll never do anything. Register for the race. Only 50 meters." But, but, I don't even have shoes, those super cool shoes with the things that poke into the track, I think they call them spikes, yeah, spikes, ok, I think I can do this. That is how I found myself on the track, in my spikes, down in the blocks waiting for the gun to go off and repeating over and over "Don't fall down, don't fall down" which I am quite sure is not a mantra recommended in sports psychology, but it was all I had. The race only lasted a few seconds and I didn't fall down; I didn't win a medal, but I finished. I knew I could do better. It would be another year before I would compete again, but this time, it would be an entirely different race, because I would be an entirely different runner.

Before that could happen, however, three things would have to occur. First, I would participate in a Spartan Sprint Obstacle Course Race, second, I would participate in a Spartan Sprint Stadion, and third, fate would intervene. I'll talk more about obstacle course racing in the next chapter, but suffice to say, it's a blast; a playground for adults. It also requires speed, endurance, strength, and agility. After completing the first obstacle course race in April of 2022, I wanted to know more about the concepts of speed, agility, and quickness (SAQ). I started reading and studying different drills that addressed those issues. I looked for classes or training, but nothing seemed to fit, so I put it aside to concentrate on training for the next race which I knew would involve running up and down stairs at a local stadium. After that race, I decided that stair running was a good way to build endurance and develop leg strength, so I kept at it. Saturday mornings would find me at the local high school running stairs with a lap around the track in between. It was there that fate would present an opportunity, if only I was brave enough to seize it.

One Saturday, after completing my workout, I noticed a man and a young, perhaps college age, woman out on the football field. I could tell it was a coach and athlete relationship, as he was directing her in different athletic drills. I watched for a bit and liked what I saw. He pushed her and encouraged her in equal measure. She looked like she was working hard, but still having fun. I thought that maybe he could help me develop my speed and agility, but if that was going to happen, I was going to have to put myself out there. You may be thinking that I was worried that I was too old or not a good enough athlete. Neither of those things entered my mind. Put me on a stage in front of a hundred people and I'm golden, but one on one, no thank you. I've been this way for as long as I can remember. As an attorney, I could use my "attorney persona" but as "just me," it's a lot tougher. Even as I write this I am thinking "how ridiculous," but there it is, so there must have been something that compelled me to pull up my "big girl pants," walk up to the coach and ask "Do you train older women?" He said something to the effect that he would train anyone who was willing to work. I told him that I was interested in speed, endurance, and agility. He said he could help with that and went to get his card. When he handed it to me, he looked me up and down and asked "Half-miler?" I laughed and answered "No-miler" but that I had done some, as in very little, sprinting and if there was a distance in which I could be competitive, I'd be interested in giving that a try. He told me to look at his website and contact him.

The card said Danny Harris OLY. Doing my research, I discovered that in the 1984 Olympics, at only 18, Danny won the silver medal in the 400m hurdles. The gold was won by Edwin Moses. Three years later in 1987, Danny would end Moses' close to 10-year 122 race winning streak. I learned that Danny's childhood was challenging and when his athletic career hit a high, he was woefully unprepared to handle it, leading him to some dark places. Danny came out of the dark places and into the light but then let his ego get the best of him and lost just about everything he had gained. When we met, he was, once again, coming back into the light.

Had I known everything before that Saturday, I might not have approached him. I don't know for sure. But since I had, I felt he deserved the opportunity to be heard. I called him and asked him to tell me his story. I wanted to know whether he would own it or try to play the blame game. How he answered would determine our future. Because you are reading this, you know how it ends.

Spike Up!

We began training the following Sunday with the goal of me competing in 5 weeks in San Diego and qualifying for the 2023 National Senior Games in the 50- and 100-meter sprint. Thanks to my regular training sessions, my body was strong, and thanks to my previous sprinting experience, I knew just enough to be dangerous, and not in a good way. The only thing of which I had a reasonably good command was my arm swing so we basically started from scratch. Drills, drills, and more drills designed to teach my body what it needed to do. In the blocks, out of the blocks. "Don't pop up, propel forwards!" "Drive, drive, drive!" "Knees up!" "Dorsiflex!" "Push, push!" "Finish, Finish!" "Loosen up!" "Not so mechanical!" "Stop thinking!" "We're playing chess, not checkers!" "Good job!" "That's it!" Over and over and over. Strange to me at the time, was that Danny never had me run a "practice race." I now understand that you can't create the feel of competition, every race is different, and you run the race you need to run; aiming for and / or falling short of a certain time (except in very rare circumstances) is a fools' game. I would go on to win gold with some of my worst times, but first, I had to get past the qualifiers. I had to "Spike Up!"

The first time Danny directed me to "Spike up!" besides thinking how cool it sounded, I thought he just meant I should put on my spikes. Yes, it means put on your shoes, but it also means bring your attitude and get ready to work. Five weeks later, when I toed the line, there was no "Don't fall down." There was silence, focus, a little fear, and yes, just a hint of attitude. I was "Spiked up." And when it was over, there were 2 qualifying spots with my name on them.

In preparation for Nationals, I continue to train (in the gym, on the track, on hills, in the pool) and to compete, and I can tell you that training is harder than any competition. I've asked my body and my mind to go further than they have ever gone before. The first time I tried to sprint 200 meters, I imploded at around 150. Hands up in surrender, I was finished, commonly known as "hitting the wall." I've since experienced what Coach calls chipping away and breaking through. It happened running 300 meters. At about 250, he could see I was starting to lose it, but I kept pushing, chip, chip, chip. He was waiting to see what would happen, would I hit or break. I broke through. Describing the physical and mental feeling of that moment is almost impossible. Your legs are shaking, it hurts to

Spike Up!

walk, and your breath is heaving. You're close to tears, not of pain or of joy, but something else. I had seen it happen with a young runner, but I didn't understand it and certainly didn't think it was something that could or would happen to me. At that moment I understood how that young runner felt, the physicality of giving everything that you have in order to achieve a goal. It's awful and fantastic at the same time because you know that you've given your best, you've finished it and as Coach reminded me "It's ok to hurt".

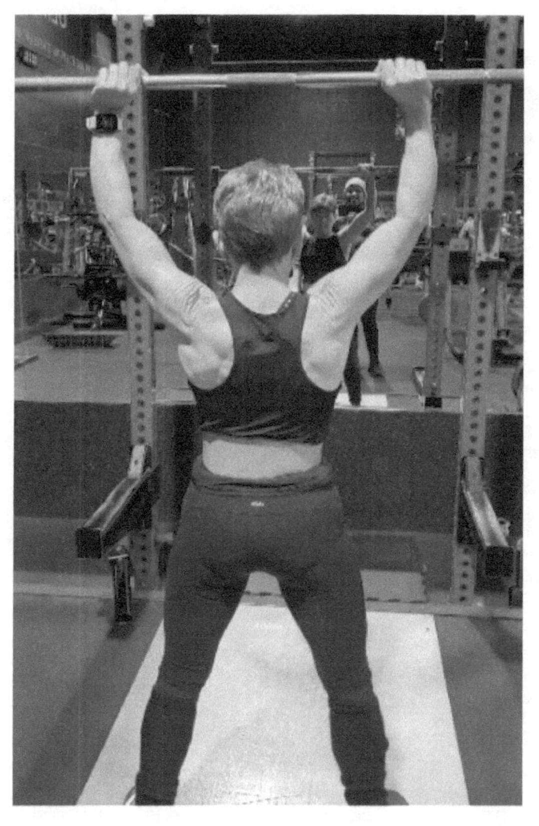

Serious time in the gym at 61

Spike Up!

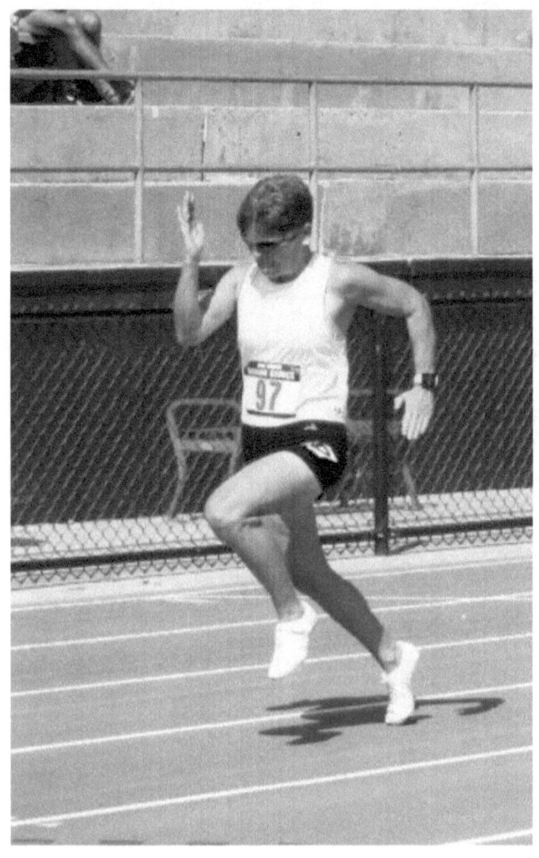

Qualifying for the 100m, San Diego 2022

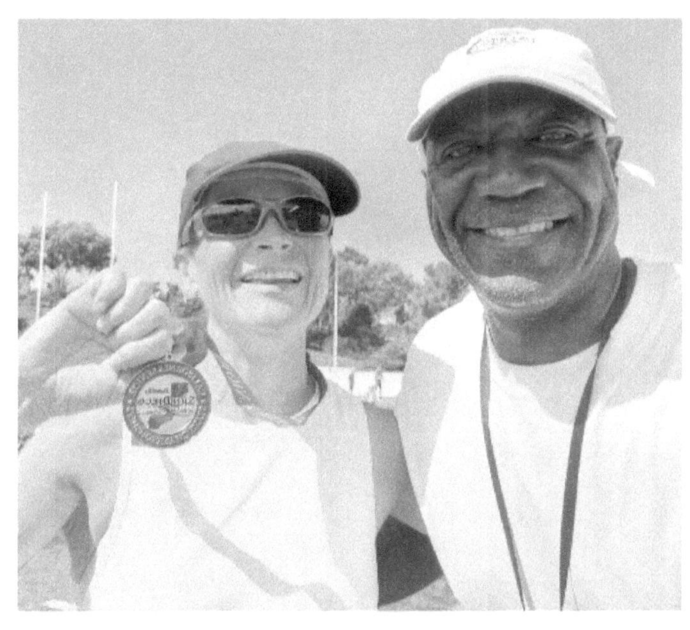

With Coach after the 100m

One qualifier down, one to go

Spike Up!

CHAPTER FIVE

Becoming Spartan

Remember when you were a little kid on the playground? You'd run around until you got tired and then you'd stop and do something else. Climb on the jungle gym, slide down the slide, go as high as you could on the swings and then propel yourself through the air. Obstacle Course Racing is a lot like that, but with special shoes that grip the ground and don't hold water.

In January 2022, Carlos told me that Karen (of Quaranteam fame) mentioned doing a Spartan Sprint Obstacle Course Race. I had no idea what that was, but figured, why not? Spartan provides a lot of information so we knew what obstacles to expect and, with the help of YouTube, had some idea how to overcome them.

Spike Up!

Whether we would be able remained to be seen. With 3 months to go, we upped our training. We ran hill trails at Griffith Park, and did special "Spartan" workouts on Saturday mornings and Sunday afternoons. In addition to pushups and pull ups, we flipped tires and raised weight plates with a pulley system; we walked uphill on the treadmill carrying sandbags; we climbed ropes and did 70 pound "farmer carries" around the gym. We were as ready as we were ever going to be, so we thought.

Pulling into the parking area at the old Fox Race Course in Pala, we could see people in the distance running up a hill. Who were they? A training group? A running team? Oh no, you have got to be kidding? Whose stupid idea was this anyway? I blame Karen. This was her idea. "Oh, I know people who have done it that weren't in great shape." What did that mean? Karen is 31. We've been training for 3 months. Carlos is 51. We're in great shape. I'm 61. I'm going to die, and I'm pretty sure there will be no monuments involved. And then we were taken over by the energy of the race. "Spartan! What is your profession?" "AROO!" And we were off.

5k and 20 obstacles later, we claimed our medals. We had jumped over walls, carried sandbags and 5-gallon paint cans filled with rocks. We ran. We had hoisted heavy objects and climbed up a rope. (I learned during training that rope climbing is my superpower) We ran. We had traversed walls using only fingers and toes. We ran. We had climbed up cargo nets and crawled under barbed wire. We ran. We had fallen off the monkey bars and the rings. We ran. We had thrown a spear and swam under a wall. We ran. We had jumped over fire. I didn't die. Wet, muddy, and tired, we were Spartans. "So, when do we do this again?"

Stadion was different. No fire and no water. There were still hoists, ropes, walls, and heavy things to carry but also more traditional exercises including jumping rope, slam ball, box jumps, and burpees holding a 30-pound tube. There were also a lot of stairs. A lot of stairs. Being pretty sure I wasn't going to die, my goal was to conquer the monkey bars and rings, both of which had defeated me, in spectacular fashion, at Pala. Not so this time. I had developed my technique and flew across the bars like they were nothing. The rings were a bit trickier, but I owned those too. Only the spear throw defeated me, again. When it was over, we were hot, sweaty, and looking forward to the next challenge. Little did we know.

The last race of the year was in Castaic. It was cold and drizzling. Dressed in layers, I was still cold. Everything was wet and muddy. I had to concentrate on every step, just to stay standing. I still swear we climbed uphill, both ways. At one point, we were so high up on a ridge, the fog blocked the view of everything below. I was miserable. Ropes remained my superpower, but the monkey bars and rings were lost causes. Carrying a wet sandbag, the thought "I can't do this" flashed through my mind. I didn't indulge it, and telling myself to "buck up," kept going. When we finally arrived at the second to last obstacle, the dunk wall, which required us to wade into cold, muddy water and duck under a wall, I looked at Karen and asked "Are you going to do it?" When she said "Yes," I said "okay, but not in all these clothes". So, we stripped down to sports bras, leggings, and shoes and in we went. Speaking solely for myself, it was not a look you would want to know better. With my white stomach, I'm surprised moths didn't swarm. But it worked. The water was freezing, but once we came out, we were able to put on dry shirts and finish the race with what little dignity remained. It was the hardest thing I had ever done. I will never do it again, until next time, when I will race age competitive. Take that Castaic!

Spike Up!

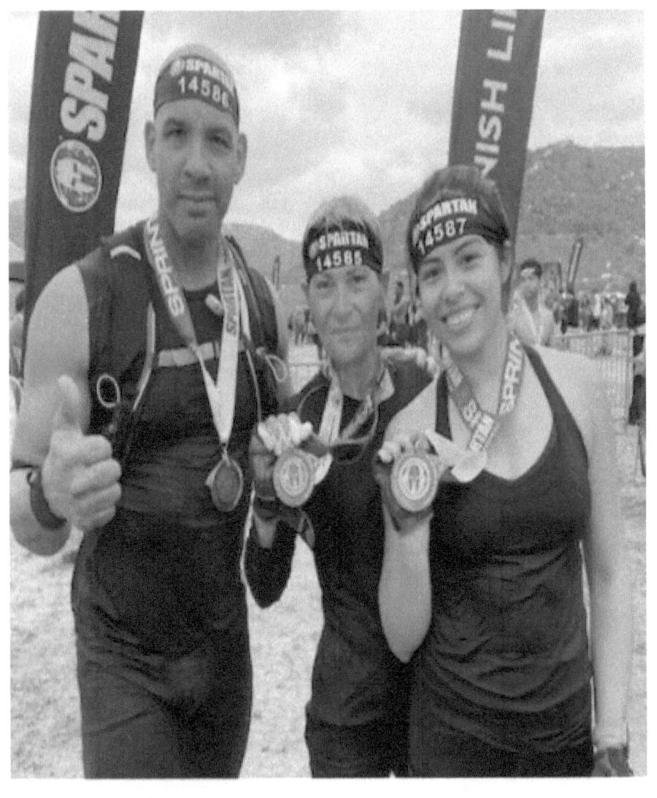

Flanked by my trainer, Carlos, and the one who got me into this, Karen

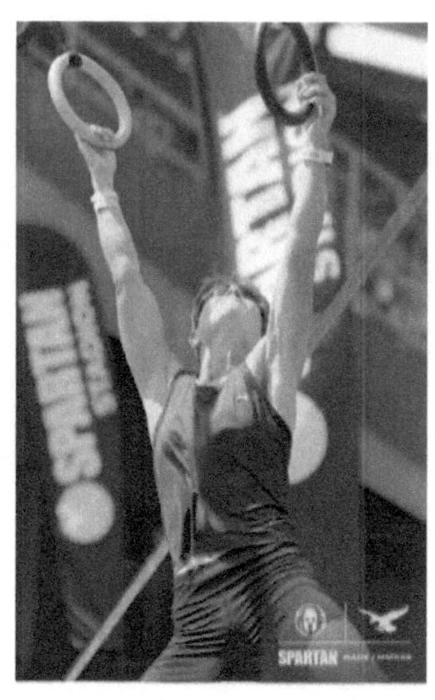

Flying at Stadion

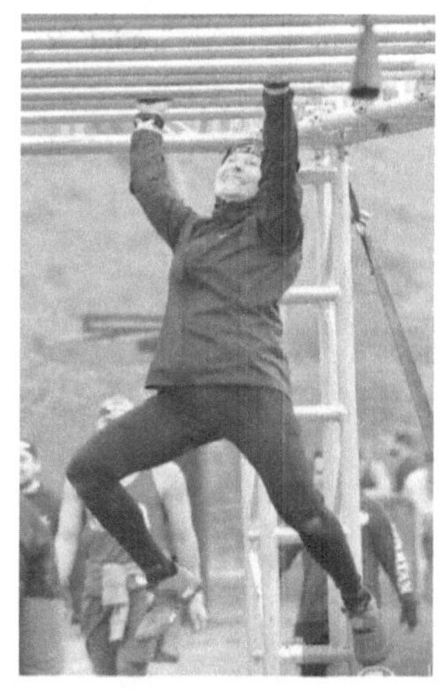

Hanging on in Castaic

Spike Up!

CHAPTER SIX

Final Thoughts

Sprinting is a singular sport. It's just you, the track and the clock. It requires technique that can only be developed through practice and a mental toughness that can push the thought of pain aside and drive you to give your very best. Obstacle course racing can be singular. If you are competing, it's you against the clock but the intensity is of a different nature and over a longer period of time. Or, you can be a part of a community of racers who are in it for a challenge, but also for fun. I want to race competitive for the experience, but I'm not sure it's something I want to do for the long term. Part of the fun of obstacle course racing is helping and cheering others on. My joy is compounded by the success of others. I love showing others how to climb the rope and am probably more excited than they are when they succeed. The mental aspect is different as well.

Spike Up!

In sprinting, pain plays a factor. In obstacle
course racing, it's fear, and it usually takes hold
at the top of an obstacle. The slip wall is one of
those obstacles. It's a metal wall at about a 45-
degree angle. There are ropes attached to the
top which you must use to pull yourself up.
Once you are at the top, you climb over, and
climb down a ladder like apparatus. There are
two challenges. First, the wall is wet and
slippery. If you don't plant your feet and lean
back, you will fall on your face and slide down.
Second, in order to get over the top, you have to
let go of the rope.

At Castaic, I was next to a racer who got stuck at
the top of the slip wall. Only a half an obstacle
away from victory, she was crouched down, eyes
closed, trembling, and hanging on for dear life.
She was terrified. Friends and strangers stopped
to encourage her, to let her know that they were
there, and that she wasn't going to fall. Letting
go of the rope, one hand at a time, to the cheer
of the crowd, she got over.

I chose to become an athlete. You can choose to
become whatever you want. Show up, do the

work, give your best. It might not be easy. It might hurt. You might feel scared. You might even find yourself stuck at the top of a wall. And if you do, know you have two choices: you can give up and slide down or you can trust yourself, your friends, even total strangers, and JUST LET GO!

Spike Up!

Afterward

Recently, I heard a writer say that if you are going to write a book with the hope that at least one person will read it, you are wasting your time. Why put all that time and effort into something that only one person might read? Perhaps he was encouraging the listener to "Think big," but his tone said otherwise, and I am ashamed to admit it, but I almost fell for it and abandoned this book. I almost let the mocking tone of a total stranger who wasn't even talking to me stop me from doing something I wanted to do with the hope that it just might give someone else the nudge to do something that they wanted to do.

Hopefully, I've given you that nudge, encouraged you to keep going, and provided some amusement along the way. If nothing else, I've learned something about myself. As I was writing, I noticed that many of the places I've gone and things I've done are as a result of others leading me there. Without them, I would never have done those things and become the person I am. Although I will continue to look to others, I will also look to myself, take my own advice and "Spike Up!"

Spike Up!

Acknowledgements

To my trainer, Carlos Guerra, thank you for your patience and support all these years. Your expertise and encouragement have been invaluable. You helped me build a body that will do what I want it to do. You told me that if I wait until I'm ready, I will never do anything. I really thought you were kidding.

To Coach, Danny Harris, thank you. Because of you, I have pushed myself further (and farther) than I ever thought possible. You taught me how to "Spike Up!" With your guidance, I am slowly learning to play chess.

To Karen Abundis, thank you for letting me be one of the "Quaranteam" and for letting me continue to train with you. If it wasn't for you, I would never have run an obstacle course race. I also wouldn't have fallen on my a** in front of a crowd or waded into freezing water half-dressed. I'm thinking I could have lived without either of those.

To everyone else, who when I said "I can't" said "You can," I thank you.

Spike Up!

To those, who when I said "I can" said "You go girl," I thank you too.

And to the annoying few, who when I said "I am the greatest," politely pointed out "No, that was Muhammed Ali," I forgive you.

About the Author

Jeanne Roy is a former prosecutor who, upon retiring from the law, jumped into the fitness world with both feet. She is a NASM Certified Personal Trainer with a specialization in Sports Performance Enhancement, a competitive sprinter, obstacle course racer and die-hard weight lifter. She loves teaching and showing older adults how to stay healthy and strong so that they can do whatever it is they want to do. She lives in California with her husband, Dean, who not only tolerates her obsessions, but encourages them.

Spike Up!

www.ingramcontent.com/pod-product-compliance
Lightning Source LLC
Chambersburg PA
CBHW021344160726
47994CB00007B/2841